MENTAL HEALTH

David Carpenter

First edition 1991
Reprinted 1992 1993
Revised 1994
Second edition 1996
Reprinted 1999
Revised 2001
Reprinted 2001

Published by
Emap Healthcare Ltd
Greater London House
Hampstead Road
London
NW1 7EJ

Companies and representatives throughout the world

Photography: Laurence Bulaitis, Richard Smith

Reprographics by
Graphic Ideas Studio
Karen House
1–11 Baches Street
London N1 6DL
Tel: 020 7608 3639

Printed in Great Britain by
Drogher Press
Unit 4 Airfield Way
Christchurch
Dorset BH23 3TB
Tel: 01202 499411

ISBN 1-84244-014-4

Contents

Introduction

The purpose of this module

This book is one of four specialist modules which form part of the Emap Healthcare Open Learning Enrolled Nurse Conversion Programme:

- *Community Healthcare*
- *Care of the Mother and Newborn*
- *Mental Health*
- *Learning Disability.*

These modules are designed to be used in conjunction with EN Conversion Book 1 and Book 2.

Each of these books can also be used on its own for professional updating, or as a reference when relevant experience arises in practice.

The *Mental Health* module and your related experience are not intended to turn you into a specialist mental health nurse. However, the experience you gain will help you to develop an understanding of the impact of mental health problems on the people concerned and those who care for them: health and social care professionals, voluntary sector providers or their families and friends.

How to use this module

The UKCC requires that, in order to register as a first-level nurse, second-level nurses (general) need to undertake a conversion programme which includes community healthcare, care of the mother and newborn, mental health and learning disability, including theory and practice.

How and when you gain your experience of mental health nursing will depend on your tutor and the relevant nursing managers. However, we do recommend that before you start on this specialist module you work through the first two Sections of the *Community Healthcare* module, which contain essential information on demography and its relationship to the provision of care.

The material in the four specialist modules contains more work than the UKCC minimum requirements specified above for first-level registration. However, you may find that by dovetailing some aspects of the project work, based on the community profile (see below), you can be working on more than one module at the same time. The student notes which accompany the Conversion Programme give more guidance on planning and managing this work.

The community profile

Throughout the four specialist modules *Community Healthcare, Care of the Mother and Newborn, Mental Health* and *Learning Disability* you will be asked to include in your community profile relevant information you obtain from carrying out the Activities. Do not confuse the community profile with your personal profile — it is entirely separate. The community profile will provide a record — a picture — of the community in which you and your clients/patients live and work, in particular:

- The people who make up the community
- Their health, social and cultural needs
- The facilities, resources and services available to meet those needs.

If you live and work in a large urban area, your community profile may represent only a part of the larger community, for example a large housing estate. However, if you live and work in a rural area, you may be able to develop a picture of a much larger section of the community, if not the entire community, such as a small rural town.

Whatever your practice setting or specialism, the community profile should become a very useful resource for you.

As the profile grows it will enable you to demonstrate your developing knowledge and understanding of the community and your client/patient group. It will also offer a point of reference to illustrate the changes which occur, especially in resources and services, and your increasing ability to understand the possible effects of these changes on you and the clients/patients you work with.

Building your community profile

Where do you keep it?

You may wish to keep your community profile in a section of your *Profile Pack*. Alternatively, you may find it more convenient to keep it in a separate binder altogether.

How do you develop it?

You are free to develop the profile as you wish, creating sections or categories which best meet your learning objectives. However, one suggestion is that you divide it into the three sections described above, namely:

- The people — the different cultural, religious and social groups, where and at what many of them work, how supportive they are of each other, in particular those who make up your client/patient group

- The health, social and cultural needs of the community — again looking at your particular group or the community as a whole

- The local facilities, resources and services available to meet those needs — for example, shopping, transport, leisure and sporting facilities and health, voluntary and social services.

You may decide to expand on these sections, sub-divide them, or create entirely different ones.

However you create it, the profile should give you the information you need to help you provide an appropriate service for your clients/patients.

A note about reflection

Many Activities throughout the book encourage you to keep a diary. You will find more guidance on using a professional diary in *The Profile Pack*. It is important that part of your diary is kept private — for your eyes only — so that you can be completely honest about what you think. Remember that if you are writing about clients or colleagues, the diary is confidential and you do not need to show it to anyone else.

ACTIVITY
diary
Write a definition of good health that could be applied to anyone in the world.

Some Activities ask you to pause for a moment and think about certain questions. Again, these will be your private thoughts, and you may wish to jot them down in your diary as well. These are important Activities, as they will help you work out your own views — so try not to skip them.

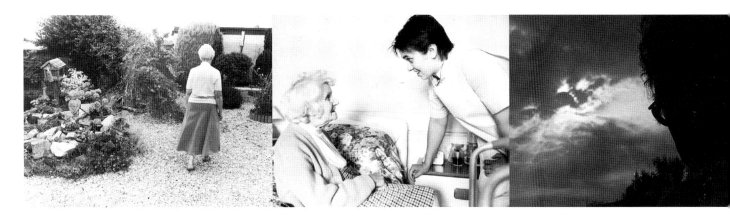

What is mental health?

Mental health is an important — and ever-changing — aspect of each individual's state of being. In this Section we examine some of the concepts on which our view of mental health is based.

Caring for the 'whole' person

Everyone's health is affected by physical as well as by psychosocial (psychological and social) factors, and nursing care is only likely to be effective if it encompasses the needs of the whole person. You may never have contemplated mental health nursing, although it is likely that in planning care in other contexts you have identified problems relating to mental health as well as physical health. There are, of course, clients who primarily have mental health problems and others who primarily have a physical illness, but nurses should aim always to practise holistically. All nurses therefore need some mental health knowledge and experience in order to:

- Plan care and practise holistically, and not treat the client as just a body in which a disease exists

- Care for a person with mental health problems who is receiving treatment for another aspect of his or her health.

You will already have some experience of dealing with mental health issues, because you will have been involved in assessing and planning those aspects of psychosocial care which are included in every client's care plan. You may not have considered these issues as directly relating to mental health, but as you will see in this Section, for most general nurses the psychosocial aspects of care are most important in determining the state of the client's mental health.

ACTIVITY
diary and community profile
Look at the care plans of three clients you currently provide care for. Make some notes in your diary on:

- Psychosocial aspects of their care which have already been planned

- How their psychosocial needs were identified, and by whom.

Does your care planning system pre-identify the psychosocial criteria to be assessed for each client, or is each person considered individually? What do you think the advantages or disadvantages might be? Think about whether it might be possible to make changes to ensure each client's needs are assessed fully. Enter your findings to your community profile.

FEEDBACK

A client's physical care needs can usually be assessed and planned using criteria which are fairly objective, that is, described and understood by everyone in more or less the same way. However, a person's psychosocial needs have to be looked at from a completely different standpoint. Assessing the psychosocial needs of the individual is a subjective process, in which your values, attitudes and beliefs are as much a part of the process as those of the client.

Health and mental health

ACTIVITY
diary

Think again about the three clients you considered in the previous Activity. Describe them in as many ways as you can that are not based on their symptoms or diagnosed illness. Your descriptions could include such things as social ties, age, or work environment — for example 'a 38-year-old unemployed father of three school-age children who was admitted as an emergency last night'.

Now use these descriptions to determine the needs and problems you think those clients have which might be psychosocially based. Compare your conclusions with those recorded in the original care plans, and make notes in your diary of any differences you find.

An individual's state of health is usually a subjective matter, based on that individual's view of what health is and what illness is. For example, how people with diabetes see their general state of health will vary enormously, depending on their personal views of health and illness. Someone whose condition is stable might see themselves as completely healthy if they feel that their diabetes does not affect their life to any great extent. If, on the other hand, they feel that the measures they have to take to keep their condition stable does affect certain important areas of their life (such as being able to eat out), then they might consider that they are not completely healthy.

When it comes to mental health, definitions are even less clear-cut. As you saw in the last Activity, assessments about a person's mental health must always be subjective, and for this reason there is an enormous amount of controversy about what constitutes mental health and mental illness. Moreover, people who have been diagnosed as having a specific mental illness often see themselves as being completely well.

What is health?

The most frequently quoted definition of health is that given in the preamble to the constitution of the World Health Organization (in: Gillan, 1986):

'Health is a state of complete physical, mental, and social well-being, and not merely the absence of disease or infirmity.'

ACTIVITY
diary

Write a sentence describing what you consider to be a state of 'complete mental well-being'. How often do you think it is possible to reach this state?

FEEDBACK

Different people will have their own ideas about what constitutes 'well-being'. You might, for example, have written 'absence of worry', or 'lack of anxiety', or you might have been more descriptive, perhaps mentioning feelings of inner peace, or 'being at one with the world'.

Maslow (1968) described the concept of self-actualisation, a state of having achieved, or of moving towards, one's full potential and reaching fulfilment. He observed a number of characteristics common to 'self-actu-alised' people, for example tolerance, spontaneity, self-reliance, independence, appreciation of small things, creativity, sense of humour etc. Rogers' concept of the 'fully functioning person' (1965), though similar to Maslow's, focused on the potential for growth rather than the once-and-for-all achievement of a state of fulfilment.

We would be surprised if you said it was never possible to achieve a complete state of mental well-being or fulfilment. However, you may have said that it is not easy to maintain a state of complete mental well-being for very long — the pressures, demands and worries of everyday life tend to act against this.

You may also have found that a state of mental well-being is not easy to assess. Fears, worries and stress, for example, can affect mental well-being but, as we saw above, most people would not consider themselves to be mentally unhealthy merely because they have a few worries. There would be a problem only if the worries were so preoccupying that they were unable to lead what they would consider to be a 'normal' life. So mental health might be a matter of people feeling in control of their own lives.

Notes

ACTIVITY
diary
What does 'being in control of your life' mean to you? Make some notes in your diary. You may find it interesting to discuss this question with other people in your life and see how views can vary.

FEEDBACK

Once again, your response to this Activity will depend on your own views and beliefs. Some people believe that they should be in control of all aspects of their life, and they blame themselves if things go wrong. Others believe that everything in life is controlled by fate, or by God, and feel that they themselves have very little influence on the course of their lives.

Rotter (1966) developed the concept of the 'locus of control', contrasting two different attitudes:

People with an 'internal locus of control' believe that their behaviour makes a difference to the outcome of situations and act accordingly to influence what happens to them

People with an 'external locus of control' are convinced that what they do will have no effect on what happens to them but rather that they are controlled by outside events and forces.

Most of us will be somewhere between these two polarities. Most people experience occasions when they feel as though they do not have as much control over their life as usual. For example, if they are seriously ill it is likely that they will be unable to do all the things that they would wish — they lose control, and this is frightening.

We could say, then, that:

'Mental health is a state of well-being resulting from a feeling of being in control of one's own life.'

If we accept this definition, we can see that everyone may have mental health problems from time to time. Even a common cold can interfere with our day-to-day control over our lives. It is well known that influenza is a common cause of depression and, although theories attempting to account for this are complex, loss of personal control, feelings of vulnerability and recognition of the fact that we have no means of avoiding the effect of a simple virus all provide part of the explanation.

Stress, too, is a very common experience that can affect people's mental health. The excessive demands of work and family life, perhaps combined with feelings of guilt at not coping very well, can lead many people to feel out of control at times, and unable to cope with their life.

FEEDBACK

ACTIVITY
diary
Try to recall the last time felt you were not in control of your own life.

What caused your loss of control?

What did you feel like? Write down some of the feelings.

Ask a friend or relative who recalls your behaviour at that time to explain the changes which occurred.

How did you regain control? Write down the circumstances (people, things or events) which helped you.

You can probably see that you yourself have experienced some problems which affected your mental well-being. The events you described in answer to this Activity would certainly represent a deviation from the WHO definition of 'a state of complete mental well-being'. Most of us experience these sorts of problem from time to time, and most of us find ways of dealing with them without too much long-term disadvantage to our physical or social well-being.

So if 'complete mental well-being' is a state which most of us seldom achieve, when does a mental health problem become a condition requiring professional intervention?

Normality and abnormality

Many people, when questioned about it, will admit that they have felt the urge, at one time or another, to jump off a tall building or into the path of an oncoming train. These feelings are fairly common and are difficult to explain, since many of the people who experience them have no immediate threat to their mental well-being at all. Even if we do feel a bit depressed, or overburdened with life's problems, most of us do not wish end our life.

So even if we lose control over certain aspects of our lives, and may feel like jumping off a high building or murdering the kids, we do not actually do it. Our thought processes ensure that feelings such as these are not translated into action. We could therefore amend our previous definition of mental health so that it reads:

> 'Mental health is a state of well-being resulting from a feeling of being in control of one's life. Control over normal feelings is maintained by rational thought processes.'

So, according to this definition, feeling like jumping off a high building or murdering the kids could be regarded as fairly 'normal', but actually doing it is 'abnormal'.

ACTIVITY
diary
Without looking at a dictionary, write down your own definitions of 'normal' and 'abnormal'.

FEEDBACK

Most definitions of normality refer to something which conforms to commonly agreed standards or levels. This is fine when you are talking about an X-ray, for example, or the results of a biopsy. In these cases standards of 'normality' are based on scientific research which gives us a measure of what you might expect to see in a healthy body, and 'abnormal' is a measure which anyone can judge against this standard.

'Abnormality' in this context is an objective measure — something which is not a matter of opinion, but which can be judged in the same way by everyone, against a standard which everyone understands.

In other areas, however, the notion of commonly agreed standards is much less straight-forward. Even some kinds of physical illness, which can be diagnosed according to standards agreed by the medical profession as a condition which deviates from the standard of a 'healthy body', may not be regarded in the same way by the person who is held to be 'suffering' from it. Diabetes, as we saw earlier, is a good example of this. It is a serious disorder if it is not managed properly. However, most people with diabetes do not regard themselves as abnormal simply because they have diabetes, and do, indeed, live perfectly 'normal' lives.

So the concept of 'normality' can be based on the opinions of individual people, even when there are technical standards by which normality can be measured. These subjective opinions are based on the values, attitudes and beliefs of each individual and can be shaped by a whole range of factors, such as their background and personal history.

Sedgwick (1982) provides another example of this. He describes a South American Indian tribe where those suffering from dyschromic spirochetosis, a disease in which coloured spots appear on the skin, are considered normal, while those who would be described objectively as healthy, that is, not having the disease, are regarded as abnormal, and are excluded from marriage.

To some extent society has conferred the power on doctors to define disease (Jones and Moon, 1987), allowing them to make decisions such as 'this person is mentally ill and not responsible for her actions' or 'he has a bad back and cannot be expected to work.

FEEDBACK

ACTIVITY
Would you use the term 'abnormal' for any of the clients you provide care for? Explain why you would/would not use the term.

It is doubtful whether you would describe any of your clients as abnormal just because they are physically unhealthy. Being unhealthy does not mean being abnormal. However, people with comparatively minor mental health problems are often referred to as abnormal. Such people are certainly not abnormal and it is doubtful whether minor changes in behaviour can really be defined as abnormal.

Describing people and their behaviour in this way is a subjective value judgement, based on our own values, attitudes and beliefs. As such, defining a person as abnormal reflects our own perception of what is normal.

FEEDBACK

ACTIVITY
diary
Reflect on your answer to the last Activity. What idea of normality did you have in mind when deciding what your answer would be?

This question is at the heart of one of the great debates in mental health — when does a mental health problem which would generally be considered normal become mental illness? For example, when do neuroses — characterised by anxiety, obsessive behaviour or phobias — become serious mental health disorders? Someone who is scared of spiders is unlikely to be considered abnormal unless, perhaps, the phobia is so severe that it prevents the person from entering forests, cellars or even bathrooms for fear of encountering a spider there.

Does mental illness exist, or is it something which is socially constructed, created by society to explain behaviour which does not conform to that which is socially acceptable? For example, Conrad and Schneider (1980) discuss how homosexuality has been seen in different cultures and at different times as a sin, a crime, a disease and a matter of personal choice of lifestyle. Gold (1973) argues:

> 'I have come to an unshakable conclusion: the illness of homosexuality is a pack of lies, concocted out of myths of a patriarchal society for a political purpose. Psychiatry, dedicated to making sick people well, has been the corner-stone of a system of oppression that makes gay people sick.'

Jones and Moon (1987) cite evidence to suggest that every disease can be examined from the social constructionist viewpoint. They do not argue that biological measurements have no reality, but that the way they are interpreted must be seen in a social context. Diseases must not be seen as exclusively social or biological phenomena, as they are both simultaneously.

Ethnicity plays an important part in the social constructs of normality and abnormality. It is increasingly used as a means of defining social, cultural and historical differences between groups of people in a multiracial and multicultural society such as Britain's (Thomas et al., 1997). Thomas et al. (1997) remark that there are potential pitfalls in categorising people into 'ethnic groupings', including the overgeneralisation of cultural attributes to specific ethnic groups, leading to stereotyping.

When making an assessment of a person's behaviour and mental state it is important that cultural differences are understood. For example, D'Ardenne and Mahtani (1989) cite the example of high levels of eye contact found in some Arabic and Latin American cultures that Europeans may find uncomfortable. Cross-culturally, notions of 'comfortable distance' between individuals vary widely and point to the need to be aware of how we frequently interpret the appropriateness of non-verbal conventions of other cultures by our own norms.

It is also important for nurses to be aware of and give due consideration to the religious and spiritual beliefs and practices of their clients. Littlewood and Lipsedge (1989) describe how aspects of religious expression — for example 'speaking in tongues' as found in

9

ACTIVITY
diary
Try to recall occasions when you may have considered a client's behaviour to be abnormal without taking into account their cultural or religious beliefs and practices.

pentecostal religions — can potentially be confused with psychiatric symptoms of mental illness. Boddy (1989) and Lewis (1971) describe beliefs in spirit possession afflicting mainly women, and known as the 'Zar', throughout Islamic Africa. The Zar spirit is seen to cause certain mental states such as depression. 'Cure' involves the victim entering in to a dissociative trance to enable the malign spirit to speak through them. In western psychiatry such behaviour and beliefs might be considered as psychotic, i.e. as demonstrating a distorted view of reality.

Mental health and disease: the debates

It is clear that some people suffer from serious impairments of mental health, but how do we describe this illness? Consider the American Psychiatric Association's (1980) description of schizophrenia, a serious mental illness:

'A large group of disorders, usually of psychotic proportion, manifested by characteristic disturbances of language and communication, thought, perception, affect and behaviour which lasts longer than six months. Thought disturbances are marked by alterations of concept formation that may lead to misinterpretation of reality, misperceptions and sometimes to delusions and hallucinations. Mood changes include ambivalence, blunting, inappropriateness, and loss of empathy with others. Behaviour may be withdrawn, aggressive and bizarre.'

FEEDBACK

ACTIVITY
diary
Look up any unfamiliar words that appear in this description and then rewrite it in your diary in your own words, so that you are easily able to understand it.

The words in the APA description are typical of the vocabulary commonly used by psychiatrists. Much of modern psychiatric care is dominated by the medical model — that is, psychiatric care based on the traditional physician-client relationship. It focuses on the diagnosis of a mental illness, and subsequent treatment is based on this diagnosis. Somatic treatments, including pharmacotherapy and electroconvulsive therapy, are important components of the treatment process (Thomas et al., 1997).

Elements of other models of care may be used in conjunction with the medical model. For instance, a client diagnosed as schizophrenic who is treated with medication may also be participating in a behavioural programme to encourage socially acceptable behaviour (Thomas et al., 1997).

This last point brings us back to our earlier discussions of normality and abnormality. Does the description of some of the symptoms of schizophrenia above actually facilitate an objective diagnosis or is it a subjective judgement, that is, an expression of approval or disapproval based on concepts of normality and social acceptability?

Szasz, a well-known 'anti-psychiatrist', claims that there is no such thing as mental illness (1970). He believes there are some people who have what he calls 'problems in living' (for example, homelessness, isolation, criminal activity), and that it suits society to give such people a label. Schizophrenia is merely one label for the problems some people have in social adjustment. It is not a disease as we normally understand the term but a fabrication designed to medicalise what should properly be understood as social deviation.

Szasz's views are vigorously contested by most members of the medical profession. However, the description given above is typical of the way that schizophrenia has conventionally been described by the medical profession, even though it was suggested that there may be a physical cause of the disease — an excess of the neuro-transmitter dopamine.

Social scientists generally view mental illness as an essentially sociological construct. They suggest that it reflects an assessment of an individual's behaviour in relation to the accepted norms of the society in which the individual lives (Smith, 1977).

Notes

The social model of mental illness focuses on consideration of the term 'mental illness' as a form of label denoting abnormal behaviour. The initial act of labelling a person as mentally ill means that all subsequent behaviour of that person will be viewed in the context of society's view of 'mad' behaviour. One of the longer-term consequences of this view has been institutionalisation, where people considered mentally ill were hospitalised, and as a result the norms of society were replaced by the norms of the hospital environment. Critics of such practices (Barton, 1959; Goffman, 1961) described 'institutional neurosis', where clients adapted their behaviours to those of the institution, losing their capacity for independence and spontaneous behaviour (Butler, 1993). Although the provision of better community care and current social policy aim to prevent institutionalisation, many argue that this process cannot be avoided within hospital settings.

ACTIVITY
diary
Have you observed behaviour by clients that could be explained by 'institutional neurosis'? Try to recall your emotional response and your actions on such occasions.

In perceptions about mental illness, the dividing line between eccentricity and insanity is often determined by social factors, so that 'nice' people (including our own friends and relatives) are eccentric, or have 'nervous breakdowns', while more offensive descriptions, such as 'mad' or 'insane', are reserved for others.

In our earlier discussions of the concepts of normality and abnormality we noted that it is important to take into account racial and ethnic differences in assessing people's behaviour. However, despite moves to community-based mental healthcare provision, a disproportionately high number of black people are admitted to psychiatric hospitals (Cope, 1989). Further evidence suggests that black people in psychiatric hospitals receive more physical treatments in the form of electroconvulsive therapy and psychotropic drugs, and that they receive and high doses of these drugs. A higher incidence of diagnosis of schizophrenia has been reported among certain minority ethnic populations living in the UK, most notably African Caribbeans (Thomas et al., 1997), and hospital admission rates for schizophrenia are five or six times higher for African Caribbeans living in the UK than for those living in Jamaica. Other studies have found that 'mentally ill' black people are more likely to be perceived as dangerous (Brown, 1999).

Several studies also suggest gender differences in diagnosis. The majority of statistical and epidemiological analyses suggest that more women than men are diagnosed as being mentally ill. For example, women are twice as likely as men to be diagnosed as suffering from clinical depression (Paykell, 1991; Gorman, 1992). Clinically diagnosed eating disorders are 10 times more common in women than men (Krahn, 1991), as is self-harm. Other diagnoses, for example those relating to drug and alcohol misuse, have an overrepresentation of men. Whether these differences might be explained by social factors rather than biological ones remains an open question.

ACTIVITY
diary
Look again at the description of schizophrenia on page 10.

Is it objective (that is, would anyone observing the person come to the same diagnosis), or is it subjective (essentially a collection of statements of approval or disapproval)?

Does the description provide scope for taking into account differences in behaviour, for example between men and women, or between different ethnic groups?

Imagine that you are a neighbour of a person who manifests the symptoms described. What problems might you experience in relating to this person? What problems might the person have in relating to you?

FEEDBACK

You may have concluded from this Activity that the boundaries of mental illness are potentially very wide. They will depend largely upon what is agreed to be normal behaviour by the majority of people in society. Once a person's behaviour has been recognised as 'abnormal', their condition can quickly come to be described using subjective value judgements. This may then be swiftly followed by the alienation of that person from 'normal' life.

Having said this, we do not wish to suggest that mental disease does not exist, nor that it is not the concern of medicine. Nor do we wish to suggest that mental health is alone in using subjective judgements — people make subjective judgements in many areas of life. However, it is important to remember that, in caring for people with mental health problems, your attitudes are as important as your skills, as this client points out:

> 'Suggesting someone is ill is better than suggesting they are bad, as they used to do. However, this is not an illness like measles, a broken leg or diabetes, and society knows this.' (Wright and Giddey, 1993)

In the next Section, you are invited to explore some of your own values, attitudes and beliefs about people with mental health problems, and to consider why it is important to be aware of these in your nursing practice.

FOCUS

Look back to your answers to Activities 1 and 2 at the beginning of this Section. Read through the descriptions you wrote of each of the three clients, and the psychosocial needs you identified, and make a note of any value judgements they contain.

- When you have done this, try to describe each of the three clients as they might see themselves.

- How many value judgements does the description include now?

- What are the major differences between the descriptions?

REFERENCES

American Psychiatric Association (1980) *Diagnostic and Statistical Manual of Mental Disorders* (3rd edn). Washington DC: APA.

Barton, R. (1976) *Institutional Neurosis* (3rd edn). Bristol: Wright.

Boddy, J. (1989) *Wombs and Alien Spirits: Women, men and the Zar cult in Northern Sudan.* University of Wisconsin Press.

Brown, D. (1999) Black people and Sectioning. *Mental Health Practice* **12**: 9.

Butler, T. (1993) *Changing Mental Health Services: The politics and policy.* London: Chapman and Hall.

Conrad, P., Schneider, J.W. (1980) *Deviance and Medicalisation.* St Louis Mo: Mosby.

Cope, R. (1989) The compulsory detention of Afro-Caribbeans under the Mental Health Act. *New Community* **15**: 3, 343–356.

D'Ardenne, P., Mahtani, A. (1989) *Transcultural Counselling in Action.* London: Sage Publications.

Goffman, E. (1961) *Asylums.* Harmondsworth: Penguin.

Gold, R. (1973) 'Stop it, you're making me sick!' *American Journal of Psychiatry* **130**: 1211–1212.

Gorman, J. (1992) *Out of the Shadows.* London: Mind Publications.

Jones, K., Moon, G. (1987) *Health, Disease and Society.* London: Routledge and Kegan Paul.

Krahn, D. (1991) The relationship of eating disorders to substance abuse. *Journal of Substance Abuse* **3**: 239–253.

Lewis, I.M. (1971) *Ecstatic Religion.* London: Penguin Books.

Littlewood, R., Lipsedge, M. (1989) *Aliens and Alienists: Ethnic minorities and psychiatry.* Harmondsworth: Penguin.

Maslow, A.H. (1968) *The Farther Reaches of Human Nature.* Harmondsworth: Penguin.

Paykell, E. (1991) Depression in women. *British Journal of Psychiatry* **158** (supplement 10): 22–29.

Rogers, C.R. (1965) *Client-centred Therapy.* London: Constable.

Rotter, J.B. (1966) Generalised experiences for internal versus external control of reinforcement. *Psychology Monographs* **80**: 1–20.

Sedgewick, P. (1982) Illness — mental and otherwise. In: Edwards, R.B. (ed.) *Psychiatry and Ethics.* New York NY: Prometheus.

Smith, D.M. (1977) *Human Geography: A welfare approach.* London: Edward Arnold.

Szas, T.S. (1970) *Ideology and Insanity.* New York NY: Doubleday.

Thomas, B., Hardy, S., Cutting, P. (eds) (1997) *Stuart and Sundeen's Mental Health Nursing: Principles and practice.* London: Mosby.

World Health Organization (1986) Basic documents: Preamble to the constitution of the World Health Organization. In: Gillan, R. *Philosophical Medical Ethics.* Chichester: Wiley.

Wright, H., Giddey, M. (1993) *Mental Health Nursing: From first principles to professional practice.* London: Chapman and Hall.

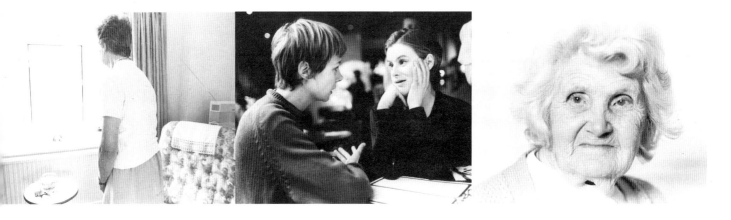

Notes

The importance of self-awareness

In this Section we look at the role of the nurse in caring for clients who have mental health problems, and consider the importance of being aware of your own values, attitudes and beliefs about mental illness. Bond (1986), Brill (1998) and Burnard (1985) examine these issues in greater detail.

The role of the nurse in mental health care

At the end of the previous Section we suggested that nurses' attitudes towards clients with mental health problems are an important factor in the care they provide. Although it is clear that nursing care involves practical, physical aspects, it could be argued that this part of the nurse's work is not the most significant. In addition to doing certain things, all nurses are also required to be certain things, for example, understanding, patient, supportive, comforting. In caring for clients with mental health problems, these 'being' aspects of the nurse's role are often more important than the 'doing' aspects.

FEEDBACK

ACTIVITY
diary
Think about the 'being' aspects of your own role. What do you think your clients need you to be? What difficulties do you have in meeting those needs?

The 'being' aspect of the nurse's role demands that you understand both what clients want and how you yourself respond to that need. This requires that you understand not only your clients, but also yourself: that you are aware of how you relate and respond to them and their condition. This is even more important when working with clients with mental health problems because, as we saw in the previous Section, the definition of mental illness itself is usually subjective, based on individual values, attitudes and beliefs.

The key to this understanding is self-awareness — this means being aware of your own values, attitudes and beliefs: 'where you are coming from', what 'makes you tick', what your 'hang-ups' are, and how these factors may be communicated to the patient, even unintentionally.

Why do we need to be more self-aware?

We have already seen that describing a person as having a mental health problem is, in essence, a value judgement. You have no thermometers or other devices to make an objective assessment of a client's mental health status. The only measure available to you as a nurse in assessing the nature of a client's mental health problem is you yourself.

It is therefore important that your idea of 'self' is well calibrated; that is, that you understand the measures you are using when you make judgements about other people.

ACTIVITY
diary
If you have a fairly high level of self-awareness, you will, for example, have a good idea of what makes you angry. Try to describe some of the people, things or situations which almost always have the effect of making you angry.

FEEDBACK

Recognising what makes you angry might also lead you to realise that when you do get angry, your anger might be out of proportion to the situation which has provoked it. If you understand that this is a feature of 'you' — that is, if you are aware of this aspect of yourself — you are less likely to fall into the trap of attributing your anger to the thing or individual concerned.

ACTIVITY
diary
Reflect on your answers to the last Activity. Can you think of any situations when your anger was out of proportion to the situation? If so, describe what happened and suggest reasons.

FEEDBACK

Understanding where your anger comes from gives you a scale, or measure, against which you can judge any angry reactions you feel in the future. This is an example of how increased self-awareness gives you a greater understanding of how you react with other people and situations.

Self-awareness in nurse-client interaction

Being aware of how you react to a whole range of different situations is at the heart of creating the effective nurse-client relationships that are so important in mental health nursing. We now explore some aspects of how self-awareness can help in situations where a nurse uses his or her 'self' as therapy, that is, where he or she is being something to help the client, rather than doing something to help the client.

ACTIVITY
diary
What do you mean when you find yourself saying things such as: 'I don't know whether it's her or me but ...'? Write one or two paragraphs in your diary, trying to explain the issues involved.

FEEDBACK

You might have suggested that the problem is simply a difficulty in understanding another person's perspective: you view something in a particular way while the other person sees it entirely differently. Who is right?

We are often tempted to believe that we are right and the other person is wrong. Sometimes we are so sure of our own opinions that we lose sight of the possibility that our own beliefs are likely to colour our description of another person or a particular situation. In fact, in some cases when we say something about someone else we might be revealing more about ourselves than about them.

ACTIVITY
diary
Think of someone about whom you have particularly strong feelings. Try to analyse your view critically. Is the person really as you describe, or is there the possibility that you might be saying something about yourself?

FEEDBACK

This Activity might have caused you to question some of the opinions you have held so far about the other person. If not, just think about the last time you complained about how opinionated another person was. Ask yourself how you described that person. Was it really in a non-opinionated way?

15

Notes

Increased self-awareness will help you to ensure that when you are describing another person, you are really talking about the person and not about yourself. For example, if you are convinced that someone else does not like you, are you really sure that it is not you who does not like you?

Attributing behaviour which is actually your own to another person is called projection. Sometimes we project a part of ourselves that we don't like or feel uncomfortable about onto another person. Anger is a common vehicle for this, and we might attribute anger to someone else who is not feeling angry at all. Alternatively we may allow ourselves to become angry at someone (even if we don't act on our anger immediately but 'go home and kick the cat' instead) when that person doesn't really deserve to be the recipient of such anger. In doing this, we are saying something about ourselves, and our reactions to certain things, rather than about the individual concerned. Understanding how the process of projection works can help us to recognise it in ourselves and others.

Sometimes we are not fully aware why we have behaved in a certain manner, and sometimes we use forms of self-deception to help us cope with negative and stressful emotions. Sigmund Freud (1901/1960) used the term 'ego defence mechanisms' to describe these processes, which also include projection. These emotion-focused strategies do not alter the stressful situation but rather change the way a person perceives it or thinks about it. We all use these unconscious defence mechanisms at times (Atkinson, 1996) because they help us over the rough spots until we can deal more directly with the stressful situation.

Freud considered repression to be the basic and most important defence mechanism (Atkinson, 1996). In repression, impulses or memories that are too frightening or painful are excluded from conscious awareness. Memories that evoke shame, guilt or self-deprecation are often repressed. Feelings of hostility towards a loved one and experiences of failure may be banished from conscious memory. For example, Pennebaker and O'Heeron (1984) found that wives of men who died by suicide were more likely to be physically ill over the years following their husband's deaths if they never confided in others that their husband committed suicide. They found that people who habitually tried to push unwanted thoughts out of their minds might find these thoughts coming back with great force, causing them much distress.

When strong mental defence mechanisms such as repression begin to break down, it is often the feelings associated with the original trauma that begin to re-emerge first, preceding any memories which might help to make sense of them. In such cases the feelings are thoroughly confusing and often frightening, and people often express that they feel as though they are going 'crazy' or 'mad'. Our need to make sense of how we feel is important and relates back to the issues discussed in Section 1 about feeling in control of our lives. It is therefore not unusual to attribute the emotional chaos to current situations, life experiences and relationships in order to try and make sense of them, rather than being able to trace them back to the original trauma.

Adult survivors of child sexual abuse often have similar experiences when they find themselves remembering past abuse that they had hitherto repressed. This often leads to serious bouts of depression, possibly requiring hospitalisation.

ACTIVITY
action
There are many other forms of ego defence mechanisms, including suppression, rationalisation, reaction formation, intellectualisation and denial. Look up these terms up in a psychology text and write a definition of each in your own words.

We said earlier that everyone uses defence mechanisms at times, and it is important to recognise when we ourselves use these processes. When we can recognise them in ourselves, we are more likely to recognise them in the people we provide care for.

Notes

ACTIVITY
diary
Thinking about your definitions of rationalisation and intellectualisation from the last Activity, reflect on your own experiences and think about occasions when you have used these as coping strategies.

It is important to remember that defence mechanisms indicate personality maladjustment only when they become the dominant mode of responding to problems. Self-awareness makes it less likely that we will misuse these strategies, and it will also enable us to help clients become more self-aware.

Another example of when the 'ownership' of feelings can get confused is when you come home feeling 'awful' but you do not know why. It is possible that the feelings you have are not really yours. Nurses can easily become 'sponges' and soak up other people's feelings. Have you ever spoken to another person who is very worried, and at the end of the conversation — although that person feels much better — you feel much worse? Taking on someone else's feelings or worries is called introjection. While such a situation might help the other person in the short term, no nurse can continue to absorb other people's problems in this way.

ACTIVITY
diary
Think of the last time you came home feeling 'awful'. Try to identify whether those feelings really belonged to you or whether perhaps you had absorbed another person's problems.

FEEDBACK

Recognising the existence of the process of introjection and whether or not it happens to you could help to avert a potential personal disaster and, moreover, will ensure that you move beyond merely absorbing other people's problems to helping them solve them.

FEEDBACK

ACTIVITY
diary
Can you think of an occasion when a client had particularly strong feelings for you? Describe what happened and how you responded to it.

This type of situation is not unusual; after all, many clients are extremely grateful for the care they receive. Sometimes, however, the feelings extend beyond this level. It is possible for a client to have feelings towards a nurse which are actually not directed at the nurse herself but at another person represented by the nurse. For example, the nurse may represent a parent who has always offered security and care, or a partner or a friend in whom the client can confide.

This process, in which the client's feelings for one person are transferred to another, is called transference. Being aware of how this situation can arise, and how you respond to it, can help you to handle it appropriately.

In order to provide appropriate nursing care, you also need to be aware of the balance of power in the nurse-client relationship. De Swaan (1990) suggested that caring encourages a dominance of the carer and a disempowerment of the cared-for. Nurses tend to need to do more for clients when they are particularly disturbed or distressed — for example encouraging a seriously depressed person to accept fluids, to have a bath and attend to their personal hygiene. When clients eventually feel more able to cope, nurses need to adapt their position accordingly and become more distantly supportive. It is important that in caring for clients we do not disempower, deskill and institutionalise them.

ACTIVITY
diary and action
Reflect on a time when you nursed a very vulnerable client who needed a lot of personal care. Did you find it difficult, as their position improved, to do less for them? Discuss with a colleague how, when the time is right, doing less can be doing more.

Attitudes and prejudices

Although many people believe that they do not hold any preconceptions or prejudices, increased self-awareness can help you to identify your own assumptions and views which may affect the quality of the care you provide.

For example, it is common to claim that smokers waste healthcare resources; they are frequently seen as second-class clients. No one is suggesting that smoking is a good thing, nor that it should not be discouraged, but should smokers be rejected (even covertly) because they waste resources? The facts of this issue are quite surprising: smokers actually save resources because they are very likely to die before they take advantage of many of the health and social care services available; moreover, smokers contribute large sums of money in taxation.

Prejudice involves making assumptions about people and attributing certain labels and stereotypes to them. Ellis et al. (1995) maintain that prejudice can be seen in many aspects of life, often in relation to:

- Race
- Colour
- Religion
- Politics
- Sexual orientation
- Marital status
- Hair colour
- Type or style of clothing
- Height
- Weight
- Age.

ACTIVITY
diary and action
Some clients are more popular with healthcare professionals than others (Stockwell, 1984). What sorts of clients do you most like working with? Try to be honest and make a list of types of clients in order of their popularity with you. Can you spot any prejudices? Discuss your list with a colleague.

FEEDBACK

Do you still believe that you have no particular prejudices? Did your colleague help you to highlight any attitudes of which you were not aware?

Our attitudes and prejudices can also affect the care we provide even before we meet a client. For example, you saw in the previous Section that clients from certain ethnic groups are more likely to be diagnosed as schizophrenic or described as violent in behaviour.

ACTIVITY
diary
Note down in your diary any advantages and disadvantages of receiving information about clients before you meet them.

FEEDBACK

On the positive side, information might help you to prepare for the clients, either by giving you an insight into particular needs, or by allowing you to reflect on your attitudes to the information you have received.

On the negative side, however, the information you receive may determine your attitude before you have even met the person. It is important to be aware that information provided by others might actually say more about them than about the person to whom it refers. Of course, there is nothing wrong with recording personal opinions and beliefs, but they should be identified as such so that the reader can be absolutely clear where they come from. We must be able to distinguish whether a piece of information expresses someone else's attitudes or whether it is a genuine record of facts.

Information provided about a client in advance may also connect with some of your own feelings, which might prevent you from working effectively with the client. For example, a nurse who has been recently bereaved might find it difficult to work with a client who has a problem connected with grief.

ACTIVITY

diary

Think of an occasion when your own feelings might have affected your interactions with a client, and record it in your diary.

FEEDBACK

Being aware of any tendencies towards projection or introjection in yourself, knowing when you are the object of transference and being able to recognise your own attitudes and prejudices will help you to gain self-awareness which, in turn, will help you to understand other people better.

Carl Rogers (1974) coined the term 'unconditional positive regard' when referring to the ideal situation in which to be brought up, that is, that a child would feel valued by parents and others even when his or her feelings, attitudes or behaviours are less than ideal. Many people with mental health problems will have a very low sense of self-worth and will not have had experience of being accepted or loved unconditionally. If, as a nurse, you can show unconditional acceptance for the client as a person, you can offer that client an extremely therapeutic experience that may lead to an improvement in self-esteem. This does not mean that you have to accept inappropriate behaviour unconditionally, but you can, in a professional way, apply the maxim 'love the sinner but hate the sin'.

The use of 'self' as therapy

Once you have a greater degree of self-awareness, it is possible to use the 'self' therapeutically. The higher your level of self-awareness, the more likely it is that you will be able to 'be' what or how your clients need you to be.

At the end of the first Section you described three of your clients as they would describe themselves — you empathised with them. Rogers (1974) describes empathy as the ability to enter the world of another as if it were your own. Empathy is important in helping you to understand a client's feelings, but it can only be really effective if you can continue to distinguish between the client's world and your own. This can be quite difficult if you are not aware which feelings are your own and which belong to the client.

Empathising with another person is a way of managing your own feelings to benefit another person. Sympathy, on the other hand, is an expression of your feelings and is not usually a helpful therapeutic tool. People are often sympathetic simply because it makes them feel better, perhaps by giving some sort of response to a problem they cannot really do very much about. That is not to say that sympathy is not offered with the best intentions, but it does very little to help a nurse understand another person's feelings.

ACTIVITY

diary

Think about the last time you offered sympathy to a client. Try to analyse your actions and motivation in that situation.

FEEDBACK

Perhaps, thinking back, you found that you were really trying to cope with your own feelings about the situation rather than understand those of the client.

Sometimes we express sympathy by recounting a personal experience which has aspects in common with the client's problem. For example, a nurse might say 'When I had my operation …' or 'When someone close to me died …', disclosing information about herself, her ideals, values, feelings and attitudes. She may also share that she has had feelings or experiences similar to those of the client (Thomas et al., 1997). This kind of self-disclosure involves respect for the client and their experiences and can be an expression of genuine empathy. Self-disclosure such as this can be effective in providing therapy, provided it is based on an empathetic understanding of how the client will receive and react to the information, rather than being simply an illustration of how someone else coped ('Look how well I coped — why can't you?').

It is also important that self-disclosure by the nurse is always for the client's benefit. Rather than using the client as a captive audience for unburdening yourself of your own problems, you need to have a particular therapeutic goal in mind, for example to show that a client's feelings are natural and understandable in the situation.

ACTIVITY
diary, reflection
Gladys Miles, a 58-year-old single woman, was referred for radical mastectomy following positive diagnosis of carcinoma. She believed strongly that the consequent disfigurement would be so severe that the treatment would be best avoided. How would you go about helping Gladys to make an informed choice? Can you foresee any difficulties in this task?

FEEDBACK

It is likely that your own life experiences, including personal contacts with friends or relatives who have been in a similar position to Gladys, would have a bearing on the help you offer to Gladys. You may also have your own fears about this or related illnesses, and these fears would substantially affect how you go about supporting Gladys, unless you are aware of your fears and able to compensate for them. If Gladys resolved not to have the treatment, you might feel particularly strongly.

Good communication is the key to effective nurse-client interaction. In the example above, it would be difficult to help Gladys make an informed choice if the nurse was unable to overcome personal feelings in order to communicate openly with her client. Communication skills are explored in more detail in the next Section, but we end this Section by looking at your own abilities as a communicator.

What sort of communicator are you?

ACTIVITY
diary
This task could be undertaken alone with the use of a mirror, but it is far more effective if you can get a friend to work with you. Make a list of emotions, for example anger, sadness, happiness, joy, anxiety, perplexity. Mime the facial expressions of these emotions to a friend, or, if you are alone, in front of a mirror.

Do your expressions vary sufficiently or could they be misleading? What are the potential dangers of misleading facial expressions (for example, some people frown when they are puzzled)?

If you can find some obliging friends, you can use this exercise to help you become more skilled in recognising emotional expressions. Take it in turns to mime the emotions and see whether it is possible to identify the emotion portrayed.

Purposeful verbal and non-verbal communication is an important part of psychosocial nursing care. As we saw at the start of this Section, in mental health nursing the personal qualities of the nurse are part of the treatment. In this context an awareness of how you communicate is a prerequisite of effective mental health care.

The following Activity is an exercise in non-verbal communication: how well do you communicate if you do not actually say anything?

FEEDBACK

While many people are able to control their verbal communication in order to hide their feelings, non-verbal communication (particularly in the form of facial expression) often tells the truth about a person's emotions. It is therefore very important for nurses to be aware of the messages they convey non-verbally, and — even more importantly — that they are able to recognise their clients' messages.

For example, a client might not necessarily express fears and other emotions verbally, but their facial expression may reveal much about what they are feeling. The skilled nurse will use a wide range of perceptual abilities in order to anticipate the needs and wishes of clients.

You may have had the very comfortable experience of communicating with another person who is really able to understand you. This skill is achieved by heightened awareness of self and others, and can be practised using the following Activity.

ACTIVITY
diary
Try to observe non-verbal communication in others — perhaps on public transport or in some other public place. Look for facial expressions (what do you think they convey? Look at body posture as well (what do you think the person is feeling?

Ask a friend or colleague to observe you over a period of time and to give you some feedback on what your facial expressions and body postures convey to others.

FEEDBACK

This type of activity can increase your powers of observation of other people's non-verbal communication, and also develop an awareness of your own personal style. Do you show emotion readily? Do you conceal what you are thinking so that others think you have few emotions?

Verbal communication can be analysed in a similar way. It is not just about what is said, but is also about how it is said — and about what is not said. A person who talks a lot does not necessarily have a lot to say! For example, a client might talk a great deal largely because of deep anxiety; similarly a healthcare professional might hide their anxiety or uncertainty by talking a lot.

ACTIVITY
diary
Describe the following objects/concepts to some friends without using your hands (sit on them to avoid any temptation!):

• A fountain

• Cornflakes

• The weather.

Ask yourself if your descriptions show that you usually choose your words wisely. Do you describe things as you see them, as you hear them or as you feel them? When you have thought about your own views on how you communicate, ask your friends how successful your descriptions seemed to them and how they would see your communication style. Compare your own views with theirs.

FEEDBACK

People tend to have different preferences in communication. For example, some people might tend to describe what cornflakes look like, whereas others will focus on what they taste like, and yet others may describe them in relation to when and where they have eaten them. By becoming more aware of how you convey information (and how you receive and 'store' it) you can not only learn to become more alert to other people's communication styles, but also to communicate more effectively with others by using language which respects their preferences.

This Section has focused on the importance of self-awareness in mental health nursing. Thinking about all the issues that have been raised will help you to increase your level of self-awareness in the context of your interactions with clients.

FOCUS

Spend about 10 minutes thinking about and writing down the things you are aware of around you, such as sounds, smells, feelings and objects; as you do so, also note down any memories prompted by those sensations.

Preface each sentence with a phrase such as 'Now ...', 'At this minute ...', for example, 'Now I am aware of cars passing'.

After 10 minutes, study your list and count:
• The number of times you stayed in the present
• The number of times you thought of future events
• The number of times you recalled past events.

Did you dwell in the future ('Now I am wondering what to cook for dinner') or the past ('Now I am thinking about the row I had at work'), or were you alert to what it is possible to be aware of in the here and now?

Look at your list again. Note down whether the things you were aware of were:
• Mainly external — for example, what was going on outside the room, or in the world at large
• Happening to you physically — for example, tired, headache, itch, hunger
• Happening to you emotionally — for example, bored, angry, alert, interested.

If you found that you focused more on some areas than others, make some notes in your diary on the steps you could take to ensure that you develop a more balanced self-awareness.

REFERENCES

Atkinson, R. (1996) *Hilgard's Introduction to Psychology* (12th edn). London: Harcourt Brace College Publishers.

Bond, M. (1986) *Stress and Self-awareness: A guide for nurses.* London: Heinemann.

Brill, N.I. (1998) *Working With People: The helping process* (5th edn). London: Longman.

Burnard, P. (1985) *Learning Human Skills: A guide for nurses.* London: Heinemann.

De Swaan, A. (1990) *The Management of Normality.* London: Routlege.

Ellis, R., Gates, R., Kenworthy, N. (1995) *Interpersonal Communications in Nursing: Theory and Practice.* London: Churchill Livingstone.

Freud, S. (1901/1960) *Psychopathology of Everyday Life.* London: Hogarth Press.

Jackson, S., Stevenson, C. (2000) What do people need psychiatric and mental health nurses for? *Journal of Advanced Nursing* **31**: 2.

Pennebaker, J.W., O'Heeron, R.C. (1984) Confiding in others and illness rate among spouse of suicide and accidental death victims. *Journal of Personal and Social Psychology* **93**: 373–376.

Rogers, C.R. (1974) *On Becoming a Person.* London: Constable.

Stockwell, F. (1984) *The Unpopular Patient.* London: Royal College of Nursing.

Thomas, B., Hardy, S., Cutting, P. (eds) (1997) *Stuart and Sundeen's Mental Health Nursing: Principles and practice.* London: Mosby.

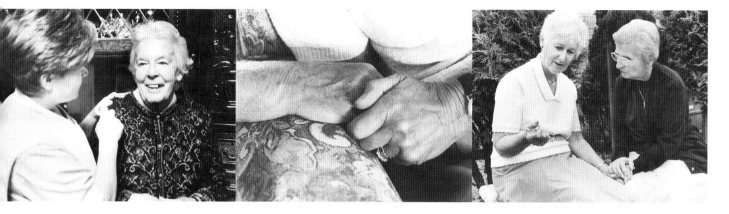

Notes

Mental health nursing skills

This Section introduces some of the specific skills and techniques which are useful in providing psychosocial care. It is important to remember, however, that simply using the techniques makes you only a technician. Nursing should extend beyond this to include a genuine therapeutic use of self, as we saw in the previous Section, by recognising that the nurse-client relationship plays a key role in overall treatment and care. Caring about your clients is an important part of this relationship.

Caring about clients

'You should not get emotionally involved with clients' is a much-stated maxim. It is often suggested that involvement is necessarily unprofessional. Professional nurses simply do not feel sad when a client is told that she is terminally ill, for example. There is some truth in this. After all, inappropriate involvement might well be unprofessional, or it might result in nurses not being able to be helpful, as their emotion could block any ability to help. On the other hand, how can nurses truly be said to care unless they are involved with the client? The key, of course, is appropriate involvement. Professional caring entails managed emotional involvement.

What is professional caring?

John Smithson was admitted to a medical ward following a serious overdose of drugs. He said that his life was not worth living since his wife had died. His only son had been killed in a road traffic accident and he had no other relatives. His life was empty, he said, and he had no particular interests and nothing to make his life worth living.

The nurse who was John's key worker felt very uncomfortable. Ideally, she would have liked to find arguments to convince him that his life was worth living but, at best, she could find only very feeble suggestions such as 'I am sure that people would miss you. Your neighbours have sent you a get-well card, so they must be concerned'.

ACTIVITY
diary
Have you ever nursed someone like John? Can you think of any way John's nurse could stop him making a further attempt on his life?

FEEDBACK

John might feel very differently about the value of his life if someone else mattered to him or if he mattered to someone else. If the nurse could really show John that she cared about him — in other words, that it would matter to her if he were to die — it is at least possible that John's life might be saved.

Sadly there is often a tendency for nurses to show quite the opposite response (that is, to think that John matters less than other clients because he has caused his own problems). Moreover, some nurses believe that if John is treated very kindly, he will be more likely to attempt suicide again. You have probably heard people calling behaviour such as John's 'attention-seeking', implying that it should be ignored or even punished. However, if John is treated in this way he will be more likely to attempt suicide again, because his belief that his life is not worth living will have been confirmed. It is more useful to consider the person's behaviour as indicating that they are 'attention-needing'.

Some nurses may believe that caring about John will do no good in the long run because as soon as he is discharged from hospital he will be back to square one and will attempt suicide again. This is not the sort of 'caring about' we mean, as it only creates a dependence which will do more harm than good.

At the heart of John's problems is probably a lack of self-esteem, of self-worth. It is not so much a case of his life not being worth living as he feels his life is not worth living. These are two fundamentally different situations. There is nothing, in the long term, that any nurse can do to make John's life worth living, but there is much that can be done to raise his self-esteem so that he is able to feel that his life is worth living. If John has the experience of being cared about, it may help him to realise that he is worth caring about. This realisation could lead to a long-term benefit and is the aim of professional caring. In extreme cases like John's, it could be life-saving.

However, many clients who experience feelings like John do have loving families and friends, as well as plenty of apparent reasons to make their lives worth living — and still go on to attempt suicide or harm themselves in other ways. Often there is no discernible reason for the self-harm, no recent life events or identified trauma. Most clients who self-harm do so not to kill themselves but as a way of coping with intense feelings — because physical pain can sometimes be easier to deal with than emotional pain (Favassa, 1989). It can be very difficult for nurses to deal with and understand such clients, especially people who repeat their self-destructive behaviour. Attempts by the nurse to understand and empathise with the client may result in feelings of frustration and impotence at their perceived failure to bring about change in and for the client. But even if nurses are unable to put an end to all their clients' self-destructive behaviour, their professional skills will still achieve some benefits for each client — even if it is just a momentary experience of being valued and cared for.

Skills for professional caring

In Section 2 you explored your own communication style, and your work on the Activities relating to this issue will have given you some insight into your strengths as a communicator. Perhaps you have also identified areas where you might need to develop your communication skills. Bear these in mind as you work through the remainder of this Section and reflect on your interactions with clients.

Listening

Listening is a necessary and integral part of communication, and care should always be planned on the basis of a partnership, with each partner respecting the other and taking the time to listen to the other.

Nurses can sometimes be so concerned with talking to clients that they can easily forget the need to listen. One of the reasons for this might be the nurse's own anxiety, caused perhaps by sincerely wishing to be helpful but actually not being sure how to.

The difference between listening and hearing

Listening is not the same as hearing. We can all easily hear what we want to hear, but when we listen we really discover things about other people.

Mrs Brown

'You seem really busy today, nurse,' said Mrs Brown, an older patient with diabetes who was due to have a below-knee amputation the following day.

'Yes, I am. The operation list is so long and as usual we are very short-staffed. It's this bug you know; half the nurses seem to have been struck down by it. You are looking good today, is that a new nightie? I expect your grandchildren will be in later — the little lad is lovely, isn't he? Oh, there's Mrs Jones calling again. I expect her water jug is empty. Nice to talk to you, I'll be back later. We'll have a chat about tomorrow. You're not too worried, are you?'

The nurse immediately went to the aid of Mrs Jones.

ACTIVITY
diary
Do you think that the 'conversation' between Mrs Brown and the nurse would have been different if the nurse had listened to Mrs Brown?

• What do you think Mrs Brown might really have been saying?

• Why do you think the nurse behaved as she did?

FEEDBACK

It is difficult to understand what went on in this interaction without knowing more details. However, you might have suggested that Mrs Brown was really asking for attention herself and was making a rather oblique reference to the fact that she was anxious about tomorrow but that no one seemed to have time to talk to her.

The nurse may genuinely have failed to pick up on this because she did not really listen to what Mrs Brown was saying. For whatever reason, she may not have wanted to get involved in such a discussion at that time, so her action may have been an avoidance tactic.

There is a huge difference between listening and hearing, and the case study also illustrates how an anxious nurse may be reluctant to give the client an opportunity to talk because of feeling unable to help.

Active listening requires you to concentrate on what the other person is saying and on how it is being said. It also requires you to be aware of your own body posture and other non-verbal behaviour, so that you are clear about the messages you are sending back to the person you are listening to.

The following Activity will help you discover how effective your listening skills are.

ACTIVITY
action
Ask a friend to talk for five minutes about family or friends you do not know. You may ask questions to clarify anything that is not clear to you. After five minutes stop and recount the information to your friend and ask whether you missed anything out.

A third person may act as an observer and give feedback on your ability to listen actively.

• What did you forget?

• How much did you remember?

• Did you find yourself being distracted by comparisons with your own friends and family or were you really able to maintain a constant interest in the descriptions given by your friend?

Starting a conversation with a client

Starting a conversation with a client is not always easy. Comments about the weather rarely lead to a mutually rewarding conversation, and topics such as politics are probably best avoided. It is clear that the first few words are vitally important in setting the scene for future interactions. The following task will help you to gain some insights into your current practice.

FEEDBACK

ACTIVITY
diary
Write down in your diary a list of the sorts of things you tend to say to clients when you first meet them or after you have not seen them for a few days. Now look closely at your list.

• Do you tend to ask questions?

Were they open, allowing the clients to expand and talk about themselves and their problems, or were they closed questions providing for 'Yes' or 'No' answers only?

Open questions allow more scope and give the client responsibilities and some control within the interaction. For example, you might use a 'broad opening' such as 'How have you been since we last met?' rather than saying 'Have you been well since we last met?'

Of course, just asking a person how he/she has been since you last met is not in itself sufficient. There is no point in asking a client a question unless you are really interested in the answer and care about the client, otherwise the question is merely rhetorical. The client is not required to answer and therefore no further interaction will follow.

Developing a conversation with a client

In Section 2 we began to consider aspects of verbal and non-verbal communication. Here we develop the theme further by considering how you can improve your communication with clients and develop active listening techniques.

Encouraging clients to talk about their concerns and their feelings requires active, facilitative listening — that is, listening to your clients carefully, suspending your own personal agendas while listening to them and demonstrating to your client that you are giving them good attention.

It is important that you are relaxed whilst listening to your client; you should not appear preoccupied or in a hurry to move on to someone else or to rush off to do something.

An open posture tells your client that you are open to what they are saying to you. If you are sitting down, try not to cross your arms or legs (or if standing avoid crossing your arms) — it can give the impression that you are not interested. Similarly, don't fiddle with things while listening, because this can give the impression that you are not interested and are anxious to leave.

If you are hoping to encourage your client to share his or her concerns with you, it is better to be at the same level, that is, if they are sitting or lying in bed it is better to sit by them. If they are standing, you should stand too. This allows better opportunities for good eye contact — although you should, of course, avoid staring at the client! It may help to lean forward slightly towards the client — but be aware of his or her need for personal space and do not lean so far forward that you invade this. Try to be aware of your facial expressions: a smile is more encouraging than a frown to help someone open up to you. Be careful, however, not to smile at inappropriate places in the conversation.

It is sometimes useful to clarify what a client has said to you if you are unsure of their meaning; this may clarify their own uncertainties too. For example, you might ask 'Are you saying you are concerned about the possible side-effects of taking this drug?' Equally, asking for clarification ensures that you understand exactly what they are trying to communicate, will help you remember and give the client reassurance that you care sufficiently to ask.

27

ACTIVITY
action
Try this Activity with two colleagues.

Person A talks about a topic of their choice for 10 minutes, person B listens, giving good eye contact and asking occasional questions to prompt person A if necessary. (Person B is likely to feel uncomfortable initially because of being so focused on one aspect of non-verbal communication.) Person C observes the interaction and makes notes on the quality of eye contact given and how person A is affected by it.

After the conversation finishes, Person A gives feedback on whether he/she felt that he/she was given good attention and was comfortable with the degree of eye contact given. Person B reflects on how it felt to give that eye contact, and person C gives Person B feedback as an outside observer.

Repeat this exercise so that each person has an opportunity to be the listener.

People often become emotional when talking about difficult problems and anxieties. Therefore it is often useful to reflect back to the client something of the content or the possible feelings that they have expressed or inferred. This shows the client that you empathise with them. For example, having listened to Mrs Brown, the nurse in the case study above might have said: 'I imagine you must be feeling quite anxious about the operation and how you will feel and manage afterwards.'

It is quite usual for clients to pause during a conversation and lose their train of thought. When this happens, it can be useful if the nurse summarises what has been said so far; the client can then resume if he or she wishes to do so.

Allowing silence

Allowing silence is often an anxiety-provoking situation for nurses. It is a skill in itself, particularly as it is sometimes difficult to assess whether the silence is beneficial to the client or not.

ACTIVITY
diary
Think back to a time when there was a period of silence during your involvement with a client and ask yourself the following questions:

• How long did the silence actually last?

• How long did you feel it lasted?

• Who broke the silence — you or the client?

• How was the silence broken?

• Did the silence appear natural? Did it appear awkward?

• Did it follow on from what the client was previously saying, or did a change of subject lead to the silence?

• Was the silence comfortable or unpleasant?

• What was the client expressing non-verbally during the period of silence?

FEEDBACK

Were you able to distinguish between a comfortable and an uncomfortable silence? If the silence was broken by you, was it because you felt uncomfortable or was it because you honestly felt that the client wanted the silence broken? Some people feel very uncomfortable with silence, but (like listening) silence shows that you care for and respect the other person.

Thomas et al. (1997) describe how silence can be used therapeutically. For example, if you sit with a client in silence, you non-verbally communicate interest and involvement. Often people who are depressed do not have the energy or motivation to talk about their problems but draw some comfort from having another person sitting with them in silence. The message the nurse will be trying to convey is 'I accept that you do not want to talk, but you are a person worthy of attention and consideration.' This can be very valuable to a person whose self-esteem is low.

Sitting in silence also allows the client time to think and gain insights, slows the pace of the interaction, and encourages the client to initiate conversation while the nurse conveys support, understanding and acceptance (Thomas et al., 1997).

If you perceive that a client feels uncomfortable with the silence, you should break it. You should also attempt to establish whether the client minds you sitting with them or whether they would like some privacy — provided, of course, that the client is not at risk if left alone. It may be that the client is shy or feels socially awkward and would prefer to answer questions rather than initiate conversation.

It is important to note that the use of silence in communication varies between cultures (Ellis et al., 1995), and sometimes within cultures. Western cultures tend to view silence in conversation in a negative way and may feel uncomfortable with it. We might believe that it indicates an unwillingness to communicate or a lack of interest. In eastern cultures, however, silence is more common and the expression of thoughts and feelings is discouraged (Ellis et al., 1995). This obviously has implications for nurses in how you might make sense of a client's attitude and tendency to silence.

Times when you might have nothing to say

We all know that not every client can be cured. Some people have diseases for which there is no cure. This can be a shock not only for the client but also for the nurse, who can be left feeling that there is little that can be done or said to help the client cope.

We have all experienced deep feelings of helplessness from time to time. If we have no answers, how can we help the client cope? We have already seen that to keep talking is not necessarily helpful; we know that we should listen, but sometimes there is no talking to listen to. How do we show that we care about a client in this situation? It is at such times that the nurse's silence might be the most beneficial course of action for the client. Silence can be an active intervention. It is not an abandonment of care — in fact it can be extremely hard work. Consider the following case study.

Mrs Peters

Mrs Peters had had a long history of intestinal problems and had recently been admitted for an exploratory laparotomy. It was established that she had widespread cancer, including liver involvement, and that no curative treatment was possible. After the surgery Mrs Peters asked the doctor to tell her what he had found, making it clear that she wanted to know the truth. The doctor was obviously uncomfortable, being aware that Mrs Peters was only 35 and that she had a young family. He told her the truth, as she had asked, and then left shortly afterwards.

It was clear to the nurse that Mrs Peters needed help, but what could she say? Were there any reassuring words that could be offered? The nurse was aware of her own feelings of helplessness and was almost frozen to the spot on which she stood.

ACTIVITY
diary
• What do you think the nurse could have done to be supportive?

• Have you ever been in a situation such as this? What did you do and what did you feel? Share your experiences with a colleague.

FEEDBACK

It is quite possible that Mrs Peters just needed someone to be with her. She knew that there were no magic answers, but it would have helped her if she had had real human contact while coming to terms with her situation.

Perhaps in considering this case study you found it difficult not to think 'What if this were me in this situation? How would I cope?' It is quite natural to identify with the client in this way, and this may be one of the reasons why some nurses avoid this type of contact — because it can be a painful reminder of our own mortality. If you can use your own fears positively, they can help you to care by putting you in touch with the client. On the other hand, our fears can sometimes get in the way of genuine caring. The important point is to be aware of what is happening and act accordingly.

Silence is a risk, because it is one of the hardest forms of communication. However, it is communication, and the non-verbal interaction can clearly communicate the message: 'You matter, I care about you. You deserve time and space. I will make no demands of you, I will just be with you'. In Section 2 we suggested that mental health nursing required being something rather than simply doing something. The case of Mrs Peters is an example of just that.

It must be emphasised that no nurse can offer support to this extent unless he/she feels supported. It is vital that all nurses and managers recognise this need for support and aim to construct networks of support.

In this Section we have considered some basic skills which might be used in providing psychosocial care. The skills may, at first glance, seem simple but you have probably discovered that this is not so. However, they are the hallmarks of the professional nurse.

FOCUS

Look back at the case studies of Mrs Brown, John Smithson and Mrs Peters.

- Do you remember any similar situations from your own nursing practice where perhaps you were not using your communication skills as well as you might have?

- Write a brief account of the situations in your diary and then outline what you would do differently now, and why.

REFERENCES

Ellis, R., Gates, R., Kenworthy, N. (1995) *Interpersonal Communications in Nursing: Theory and practice.* London: Churchill Livingstone.

Favassa, A. (1989) Why patients mutilate themselves. *Hospital and Community Psychiatry* 4: 2, 136–147.

Thomas, B., Hardy, S., Cutting, P. (eds) (1997) *Stuart and Sundeen's Mental Health Nursing: Principles and practice.* London: Mosby.

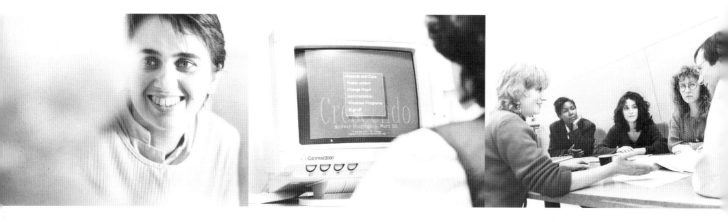

Notes

Professional aspects of mental health nursing

This Section focuses on the structures in which mental health nursing takes place and on the impact of professional and policy developments on the provision of mental health services.

The development of mental health nursing

Here we examine the organisational and structural factors that have shaped the development of mental health nursing in Britain in recent decades. *A Hospital Plan for England and Wales* (DHSS, 1962) outlined the development of a range of community alternatives to long-stay hospital care, but these were slow to materialise. A decade after the plan was published, concerns were being expressed that community care was not working (Thomas et al., 1997). However, another 15 years later, in 1987, the then Health minister Baroness Trumpington stated: 'Our policy is not to close hospitals, our policy is to build up alternative services and only then to close hospitals that are no longer needed' (Thomas et al., 1997).

One of the most significant factors that inhibited the development of community-based services was finance. Community services were intended to be developed with money that would be saved as a result of closing the large Victorian asylums, but that money was required to keep hospitals running until alternative services were available.

The NHS and Community Care Act 1990 (HMSO, 1990) tried to address this, but problems with community care have continued and have led to a series of high-profile cases. On 17 December 1992 Jonathan Zeto was fatally stabbed by Christopher Clunis, who suffered from schizophrenia, on a London Underground platform. Two weeks later another psychiatric patient, Ben Silcock, climbed into a lion's cage at London Zoo and was badly injured.

> **ACTIVITY**
> **action**
> The Sainsbury Centre for Mental Health aims to improve the quality of life for people with severe mental health problems. It seeks to influence policy and practice through a co-ordinated programme of research and evaluation, communication and development. It has produced an executive briefing paper on the New Mental Health Strategy: Modernising Mental Health Services. Use the internet (http://www.sainsburycentre.org.uk) or visit your local medical library to find and read this short document and write brief notes on its main provisions.

Public concern about the dangers people with mental illnesses present to others, and about the risk they pose to themselves, along with the evidence of related service breakdowns are some of the reasons behind the government White Paper *Modernising Mental Health Services: Sound, safe and supportive* (DoH, 1998). This is likely to set the agenda for mental health for the next 10–15 years at least.

The National Service Framework for Mental Health (DoH, 1999) fleshes out the policies of the 1998 White Paper. It spells out national standards for mental health, what they aim to achieve, how they should be developed and delivered and how performance will be measured in every part of the country.

The programme of national service frameworks (NSFs) is part of the Government's agenda to drive up quality and reduce unacceptable variations in health and social services. Government policy outlines change in three areas:

- Setting quality standards through the National Institute for Clinical Excellence (NICE) and national service frameworks

- Delivering quality standards through clinical governance, lifelong learning and professional self-regulation

- Monitoring quality standards through the Commission for Health Improvement, National Framework for Assessing Performance and an annual survey of clients' experiences of the health service.

> **ACTIVITY**
> **action**
> The National Service Framework for Mental Health sets national standards and defines service models for promoting mental health and treating mental illness in the following areas:
>
> - Mental health promotion
> - Primary care and access to services
> - Effective services for people with severe mental illness
> - Caring about carers
> - Preventing suicide.
>
> Using the internet (http://www.doh.gov.uk/nsf/mentalhealth.htm) or a library, find and read the NSF for mental health and make notes on the five areas above.

Clinical governance

Clinical governance is a framework designed to help clinicians, including nurses, continuously to improve quality and safeguard standards of care. Although the name is new, clinical governance includes many things which are already familiar to nurses, for example clinical audit, risk management, evidence-based practice, patient input and feedback, clinical supervision, continuing professional development and reflective practice. Clinical governance builds on and links together these varied activities to help promote and improve standards of care to clients.

For patients, clinical governance has put in place more explicit frameworks to assure the quality of care they receive. This includes opportunities for involvement in decision-making about their care, clear channels through which to voice their views, concerns and complaints, and assurance that these will be acted upon.

Healthcare quality

Many people have limited knowledge and understanding of the quality of the healthcare they receive — even though they may be very discerning consumers of goods and services in other areas of their lives.

> **ACTIVITY**
> **action**
> Consider the following two advertisements for acne treatment.
>
> 'Spotless' is the new miracle acne cure guaranteed to clear up problem complexions in just three weeks. Dermatologists and beauticians swear by it.
>
> 'Acnegone' ointment has been proven in several clinical trials to visibly reduce the severity of acne in sufferers with a mild to moderate condition. Side-effects are unlikely, but may occur in 0.5% of cases. 'Acnegone' should be used only after consultation with your GP.
>
> - Which preparation would you favour and why? Write notes on each advertisement, including a list of further questions you would like to pose to the respective manufacturers.

FEEDBACK

You were probably concerned to know that the product is safe and that it has undergone thorough testing to ensure safety and to ascertain its effectiveness. You would want to buy the best product based on the best available information or evidence.

Notes

Similarly, as nurses we want to provide care of the best possible quality, based on the evidence of best clinical practice. This is why the Government and the medical and allied professions are so keen to ensure that care and treatment are evidence-based.

What is evidence-based practice?

Evidence-based healthcare is the 'integration of best research evidence with clinical expertise and patient values' (Sackett et al., 2000). The process to ensure that our practice is evidence-based usually begins with an analysis of a work-based problem or issue from varying perspectives. Take, for example, the issue of nurses undertaking risk assessment. The issue can be considered from a number of perspectives:

- A social perspective: which sociodemographic factors are likely to exacerbate risk?

- A political perspective: is the local suicide rate dropping in line with national targets? How can nurses best predict risk?

- A professional perspective: which of the mental health professional groups is best placed to assess risk?

- A legal perspective: when a client detained under the Mental Health Act 1983 is granted leave to go home 'at the nurse's discretion', which factors should the nurse consider in arriving at a decision?

- An economic perspective: how much does it cost the service when a client is admitted because they were wrongly assessed as being a high risk?

- An ethical perspective: is it ethical to prevent a client from killing him- or herself?

ACTIVITY
diary
Justin Kemp, 24, has been admitted to an acute mental health admission ward with a diagnosis of schizophrenia. He frequently leaves the ward to go to the pub and arrives back drunk. Sometimes he behaves in a verbally abusive manner to staff, but on other occasions he will go to bed and 'sleep it off'. Staff are unable to give him his prescribed medication because it is contra-indicated with alcohol.

Substance misuse is a common problem among mental health in-patients. Try to analyse this problem from different perspectives, as described above.

This list is not exhaustive.

From problem to solution

Sackett et al. summarise the essential steps in the emerging science of evidence-based practice:

'Step 1 — converting the need for information — into an answerable question [that is, to formulate the problem]

Step 2 — tracking down the best evidence with which to answer that question [this may come from the clinical examination, the diagnostic laboratory, published literature or other sources]

Step 3 — critically appraising that evidence for its validity (closeness to the truth), impact (size of the effect), and applicability (usefulness in our clinical practice)

Step 4 — integrating the critical appraisal with our clinical expertise and with our patient's unique biology, values and circumstances

Step 5 — Evaluating our effectiveness and efficiency in executing steps 1–4 and seeking ways to improve them both for next time' (Sackett et al., 2000: 2–3).

Notes

FEEDBACK

ACTIVITY
diary
Drawing on your own experience of caring for a person with a mental health problem, ask yourself how much of what you do is based on evidence and how much might be custom and practice (not based on evidence)? Discuss this with a colleague.

You might find it helpful to read more about clinical governance. See for example:

Royal College of Nursing (2000) *Clinical Governance: How nurses can get involved*. London: RCN.

The Wisdom Centre (2000) A Resource Pack for Clinical Governance. Sheffield: Wisdom Centre for Networked Learning. (http://www.shef.ac.uk/uni/projects/wrp/clingov.html)

United Kingdom Council for Nursing, Midwifery and Health Visiting (2000) Professional Self-regulation and Clinical Governance. London: UKCC.

Legal aspects of mental health nursing

Admission and treatment: The role of the Mental Health Act 1983

It is a commonly held but largely mistaken belief that the Mental Health Act 1983 (HMSO, 1983) is primarily intended to facilitate treatment and hospitalisation where clients refuse such measures. It could be argued, however, that the Act is designed to ensure that the rights of people with mental illnesses are protected, as it makes clear provision for informal admission to hospital for treatment (Section 131). (Previous legislation had required clients to be certified in order to gain admission and treatment.) The Act also makes it clear that informal clients have the same status as other hospital patients: they can consent to or refuse treatment and they can leave hospital if they wish.

The nature of mental illness, particularly serious illness, is such that some clients who might most benefit from hospital admission and treatment are the least likely to seek admission (i.e. some clients, because of their illness, lack the necessary insight to seek care and treatment). To ensure ill people gain access to treatment the Mental Health Act provides facility for:

- Admission for assessment (Section 2)

- Admission for treatment (Section 3)

- Detention of an informal patient (Section 5.2: doctor's holding power; Section 5.4: nurse's holding power)

- Treatment where the client is unable to consent (Part 4).

The Act also protects the rights of detained patients by providing access to mental health review tribunals which make an independent review of alleged unjustified detention in hospital. Furthermore, detained patients are visited by members of the Mental Health Act Commission, who review the operation of the Act and ensure that clients' rights are respected.

ACTIVITY
action
The above summary gives a brief overview of the Mental Health Act 1983. Take this opportunity to read about the Act in more detail. An excellent account of the Mental Health Acts of the United Kingdom and Eire is provided by Killen (1987).

Part 3 of the Mental Health Act is concerned with the treatment and care of clients who are also subject to criminal proceedings.

The role of nurses

Having explored some of the practical and policy issues relating to care provision for people with mental health problems, we now consider the implications for nursing as a profession, and for adult nurses in particular.

While the roles of adult and mental health nurses may have been very different some 60 years ago, they became increasingly similar after the 1940s. Mental health nurses were no longer seen as 'lunatic attendants' caring for the 'insane' but rather as professionals caring for people who are ill and need treatment (Thomas et al., 1997; Davison and Neale, 1986).

In the 1980s it looked as though mental health nurses were losing their nursing identity and becoming practitioners with a therapeutic orientation. Since the 1990s they have been engaged more in caring for people with serious and disabling mental health problems, and now some people argue that mental health nurses have more in common with other colleagues practising in the mental health field (for example, social workers, psychologists and occupational therapists) than with nurses practising in other branches of nursing.

So what do mental health nurses do? The following case studies may help you to understand the role of the mental health nurse.

> James Smith complained of an increasing lack of concentration. He felt lifeless and purposeless, despite having a successful career as a draughtsman. He denied that there were any problems in his life; indeed, he claimed that many would envy his successful social situation. However, he was aware that something was amiss but did not know where to start in trying to sort out the problem.
>
> Although Robert Briggs did not have a particularly eventful sex life, he was convinced that he was HIV-positive and demanded a test. Robert had had a brief homosexual relationship in late adolescence but there had been no penetrative intercourse. By now he had a steady heterosexual relationship but was evading his girlfriend's hints about marriage because of his belief that he was HIV-positive.

Clients such as James Smith and Robert Briggs are unlikely to require in-patient treatment, but they may benefit from individual counselling within the framework of an effective nurse-client relationship. They might be referred directly to a community psychiatric nurse, as is increasingly happening, partly in recognition of the wide range of skilled intervention which many mental health nurses are able to offer.

There are now many examples of autonomous practice in mental health nursing; referrals are often made to a team of practitioners, and the team member most able to help the particular client takes responsibility for the case. This approach does not mean that the client is denied access to other team members (for example, if James were found to be suffering from serious depressive illness, it would be clear that he would require medical help and his case would be referred on).

It is often suggested that there are three main aspects to the mental health nurse's role:

- Custodial, where the emphasis is on accommodating clients with mental health problems in safety, either for the benefit of the client or in the interests of other members of society

- Procedural, including largely the provision of basic nursing care (for example, giving injections)

- Therapeutic, where the nurse is directly involved in the treatment of a client with mental health problems, either through the management of a therapeutic relationship, or by using specific therapeutic techniques, such as counselling and psychotherapy. It should be emphasised that the nurse is not necessarily a counsellor, though counselling approaches might be within the context of the nurse-client relationship. The development of this role is clearly explained by Reynolds and Cormack (1990).

Notes

ACTIVITY
diary
Discuss the above analysis of the mental health nurse's role with an experienced mental health nurse, noting in particular the changing emphasis of these three aspects over the past 10 years.

- Do you see any differences between this role analysis of mental health nurses and the role of other branches of nursing?

FEEDBACK

This role analysis can also be applied to the other branches of nursing. Custodial care was common in all branches of nursing in the past (consider, for example, the role of the nurse in the care of clients with chronic disabilities and those suffering from infectious disease before the advent of antibiotic drugs). Similarly, there is evidence to suggest that other branches of nursing are developing a therapeutic orientation in terms of the psychosocial and other aspects of their role.

Responsibilities in mental health nursing

Mental health nurses often also become involved with clients' families, and this sometimes brings considerable responsibilities. Consider the case study below.

Tony Drummond asked for help at an alcohol advice centre. He was quite clear that, although he was not an alcoholic, he tended to drink heavily when under stress and then become violent towards his wife and children. He was seriously worried that his family was at risk.

ACTIVITY
diary
Imagine that Tony had mentioned his problems to a nurse.

- What do you think a nurse should do when confronted with such a problem?

Tony sought help because he was concerned his drinking and violence put his wife and family at risk.

- What form do you think this help should take?

FEEDBACK

Tony said that he was not an alcoholic. It is likely that he was reluctant to call himself an alcoholic partly because he feared rejection by friends, family and professionals and partly because he did not see himself as fitting into the stereotype of a 'drunken down and out'. However, in admitting that he had a problem, Tony had already crossed the first hurdle.

In Tony's case, the nurse is probably unable to offer any long-term solutions and further help should be sought from other health professionals. He could well have benefited from specialist help available through either the health service or the voluntary sector. In the initial stages it would be crucial to ensure that Tony was not judged and that the trust he had invested by asking for help was respected. It is also important to ensure that, while Tony receives help to change his behaviour, his wife and children are safe. This might mean liaising with professionals outside the health service, following relevant guidelines as appropriate.

FEEDBACK

ACTIVITY
community profile
• What are the prevalent attitudes in your area of work towards people with alcohol problems?

• Does the stereotype prevail or are people willing to admit that this is a problem that can affect anyone?

• Are there any special policies in your area regarding the management of staff with alcohol problems?

Take advantage of this opportunity to learn more about the work of Alcoholics Anonymous and other support services in your own area.

Gather information from as many local sources as you can to help you carry out this Activity and record your findings in your community profile.

People who have alcohol- or drug-related problems nearly always require the combined expertise of professional staff from both general and mental health services, as well as help from voluntary organisations. You will probably have discovered this situation when investigating your own area.

Summary

In this section we have considered the roles and responsibilities of mental health nurses in their structural, organisational and legal contexts. We have focused on developments which seek to ensure the highest possible quality of mental health care, based on the best available evidence, and have placed the role of the mental health nurse within the wider context of health and social care services.

FOCUS

Look back on your notes from the first Activity in Section 1, where you considered the care plans of three clients (or, if you prefer, think about three different clients. Reflecting on your work in this module, identify any changes in these clients' psychosocial care which you would now consider to be appropriate and explain your reasons.

• Do the care plans take into account best evidence?

Bear in mind also what you have learned about the therapeutic use of self, about communication, and the structural and organisational context in which you provide care.

REFERENCES

Davison, G.C., Neale, J.M. (1986) *Abnormal Psychology: An experimental clinical approach.* Chichester: Wiley.

Department of Health and Social Security (1962) *A Hospital Plan for England and Wales.* London: HMSO.

Department of Health (1998) *Modernising Mental Health Services: Safe, sound and supportive?* London: The Stationery Office.

Department of Health (1999) *National Service Framework for Mental Health.* London: The Stationery Office.

Her Majesty's Stationery Office (1983) *The Mental Health Act 1983.* London: HMSO.

Her Majesty's Stationery Office (1990) *NHS and Community Care Act.* London: HMSO.

Killen, S. (1987) In: Wright, H., Giddey, M. *Mental Health Nursing.* London: Mosby.

Reynolds, W., Cormack, D. (eds) (1990) *Psychiatric and Mental Health Nursing.* London: Chapman and Hall.

Royal College of Nursing (2000) *Clinical Governance: How nurses can get involved.* London: RCN.

Sackett, D.L., Straus, S.E., Richardson, W.S. et al. (2000) *Evidence-based Medicine: How to practise and teach EBM* (2nd edn). Edinburgh: Churchill Livingstone.

Thomas, B., Hardy, S., Cutting, P. (eds) (1997) *Stuart and Sundeen's Mental Health Nursing: Principles and practice.* London: Mosby.

The Wisdom Centre (2000) *A Resource Pack for Clinical Governance.* Sheffield: Wisdom Centre for Networked Learning. (http://www.shef.ac.uk/uni/projects/wrp/clingov.html)

United Kingdom Council for Nursing, Midwifery and Health Visiting (2000) *Professional Self-regulation and Clinical Governance.* London: UKCC.

Notes